FALCON

BEAVER

DEER

WOODPECKER

SALMON

BROWN BEAR

C000009024

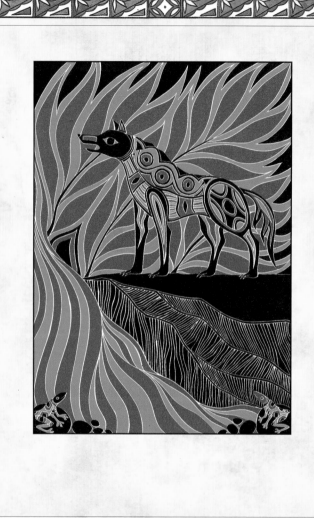

THE LITTLE LIBRARY OF EARTH MEDICINE

WOLF

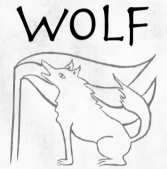

Kenneth Meadows

Illustrations by Jo Donegan

DORLING KINDERSLEY

LONDON • NEW YORK • SYDNEY • MOSCOW

A DORLING KINDERSLEY BOOK

Managing editor: Jonathan Metcalf
Managing art editor: Peter Cross
Production manager: Michelle Thomas

The Little Library of Earth Medicine was
produced, edited and designed by
GLS Editorial and Design
Garden Studios, 11-15 Betterton Street
London WC2H 9BP

GLS Editorial and Design
Editorial director: Jane Laing
Design director: Ruth Shane
Project designer: Luke Herriott
Editors: Claire Calman, Terry Burrows, Victoria Sorzano

Additional illustrations: Roy Flooks 16, 17, 31; John Lawrence 38
Special photography: Mark Hamilton
Picture credits: American Natural History Museum 8-9, 12, 14-15, 32

First published in Great Britain in 1998
by Dorling Kindersley Limited
9 Henrietta Street, London WC2E 8PS

2 4 6 8 10 9 7 5 3 1

A CIP catalogue record for this book is available from the British Library

UK ISBN 0 7513 0525 1   AUSTRALIAN ISBN 1 86466 042 2

Reproduced by Kestrel Digital Colour Ltd, Chelmsford, Essex
Printed and bound in Hong Kong by Imago

CONTENTS

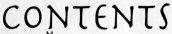

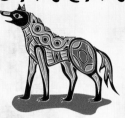

INTRODUCING
EARTH MEDICINE

TO NATIVE AMERICANS, MEDICINE IS NOT AN EXTERNAL SUBSTANCE BUT AN INNER POWER THAT IS FOUND IN BOTH NATURE AND OURSELVES.

Earth Medicine is a unique method of personality profiling that draws on Native American under-standing of the Universe, and on the principles embodied in sacred Medicine Wheels.

Native Americans believed that spirit, although invisible, permeated Nature, so that everything in Nature was sacred. Animals were perceived as acting as

messengers of spirit. They also appeared in waking dreams to impart power known as "medicine". The recipients of such dreams honoured the animal species that appeared to them by rendering their images on ceremonial and everyday artefacts.

NATURE WITHIN SELF

Native American shamans – tribal wisemen – recognized similarities between the natural forces prevalent during the seasons and the characteristics of those born

Shaman's rattle

Shamans used rattles to connect with their inner spirit. This is a Tlingit shaman's wooden rattle.

> "Spirit has provided you with an opportunity to study in Nature's university." *Stoney teaching*

during corresponding times of the year. They also noted how personality is affected by the four phases of the Moon – at birth and throughout life – and by the continual alternation of energy flow, from active to passive. This view is encapsulated in Earth Medicine, which helps you to recognize how the dynamics of Nature function within you and how the potential strengths you were born with can be developed.

Animal ornament

To the Anasazi, who carved this ornament from jet, the frog symbolized adaptability.

MEDICINE WHEELS

Native American cultural traditions embrace a variety of circular symbolic images and objects. These sacred hoops have become known as Medicine Wheels, due to their similarity to the spoked wheels of the wagons that carried settlers into the heartlands of once-Native American territory. Each Medicine Wheel showed how different objects or qualities related to one another within the context of a greater whole, and how different forces and energies moved within it.

One Medicine Wheel might be regarded as the master wheel because it indicated balance within Nature and the most effective way of achieving harmony with the Universe and ourselves. It is upon this master Medicine Wheel (see pp.10–11) that Earth Medicine is structured.

Feast dish

Stylized bear carvings adorn this Tlingit feast dish. To the American Indian, the bear symbolizes strength and self-sufficiency.

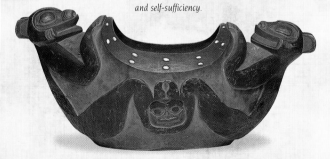

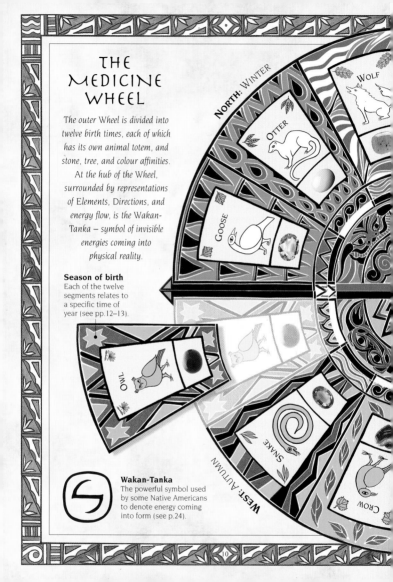

THE MEDICINE WHEEL

The outer Wheel is divided into twelve birth times, each of which has its own animal totem, and stone, tree, and colour affinities.

At the hub of the Wheel, surrounded by representations of Elements, Directions, and energy flow, is the Wakan-Tanka – symbol of invisible energies coming into physical reality.

Season of birth
Each of the twelve segments relates to a specific time of year (see pp.12–13).

Wakan-Tanka
The powerful symbol used by some Native Americans to denote energy coming into form (see p.24).

NORTH: WINTER

WEST: AUTUMN

WOLF

OTTER

GOOSE

OWL

SNAKE

CROW

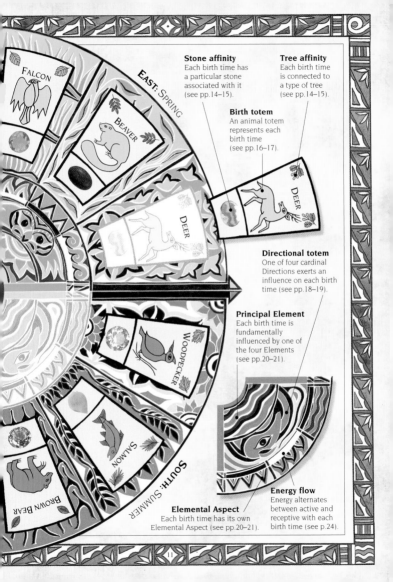

Stone affinity
Each birth time has a particular stone associated with it (see pp.14–15).

Tree affinity
Each birth time is connected to a type of tree (see pp.14–15).

Birth totem
An animal totem represents each birth time (see pp.16–17).

Directional totem
One of four cardinal Directions exerts an influence on each birth time (see pp.18–19).

Principal Element
Each birth time is fundamentally influenced by one of the four Elements (see pp.20–21).

Energy flow
Energy alternates between active and receptive with each birth time (see p.24).

Elemental Aspect
Each birth time has its own Elemental Aspect (see pp.20–21).

EAST: SPRING

SOUTH: SUMMER

FALCON

BEAVER

DEER

DEER

WOODPECKER

SALMON

BROWN BEAR

THE TWELVE
BIRTH TIMES

THE STRUCTURE OF THE MEDICINE WHEEL IS BASED
UPON THE SEASONS TO REFLECT THE POWERFUL
INFLUENCE OF NATURE ON HUMAN PERSONALITY.

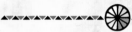

The Medicine Wheel classifies human nature into twelve personality types, each corresponding to the characteristics of Nature at a particular time of the year. It is designed to act as a kind of map to help you discover your strengths and weaknesses, your inner drives and instinctive behaviours, and your true potential.

The four seasons form the basis of the Wheel's structure, with the Summer and Winter solstices and the Spring and Autumn equinoxes marking each season's passing. In Earth Medicine,

each season is a metaphor for a stage of human growth and development. Spring is likened to infancy and the newness of life; and Summer to the exuberance of youth and rapid development. Autumn represents the fulfilment that mature adulthood brings, while Winter symbolizes the accumulated wisdom that can be drawn upon in later life.

Each seasonal quarter of the Wheel is further divided into three periods, making twelve time segments altogether. The time of your birth determines the direction from which

Seasonal rites
Performers at the Iroquois mid-Winter ceremony wore masks made of braided maize husks. They danced to attune themselves to energies that would ensure a good harvest.

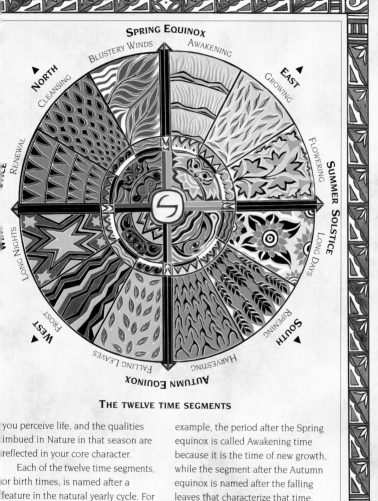

THE TWELVE TIME SEGMENTS

you perceive life, and the qualities imbued in Nature in that season are reflected in your core character.

Each of the twelve time segments, or birth times, is named after a feature in the natural yearly cycle. For example, the period after the Spring equinox is called Awakening time because it is the time of new growth, while the segment after the Autumn equinox is named after the falling leaves that characterize that time.

THE SIGNIFICANCE OF
TOTEMS

NATIVE AMERICANS BELIEVED THAT TOTEMS — ANIMAL SYMBOLS — REPRESENTED ESSENTIAL TRUTHS AND ACTED AS CONNECTIONS TO NATURAL POWERS.

A totem is an animal or natural object adopted as an emblem to typify certain distinctive qualities. Native Americans regarded animals, whose behaviour is predictable, as particularly useful guides to categorizing human patterns of behaviour.

A totem mirrors aspects of your nature and unlocks the intuitive knowledge that lies beyond the reasoning capacity of the intellect. It may take the form of a carving or moulding, a pictorial image, or a token of fur, feather, bone, tooth, or claw. Its presence serves as an immediate link with the energies it represents. A totem is therefore more effective than a glyph or symbol as an aid to comprehending non-physical powers and formative forces.

PRIMARY TOTEMS

In Earth Medicine you have three primary totems: a birth totem, a Directional totem, and an Elemental totem. Your *birth totem* is the embodiment of core characteristics that correspond with the dominant aspects of Nature during your birth time.

Symbol of strength
The handle of this Tlingit knife is carved with a raven and a bear head, symbols of insight and inner strength.

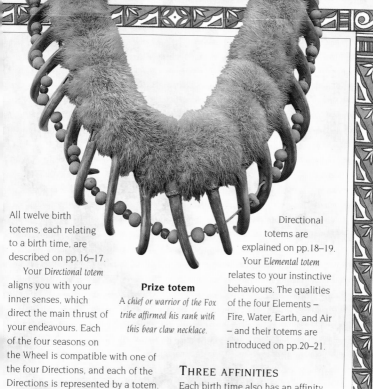

All twelve birth totems, each relating to a birth time, are described on pp.16–17.

Your *Directional totem* aligns you with your inner senses, which direct the main thrust of your endeavours. Each of the four seasons on the Wheel is compatible with one of the four Directions, and each of the Directions is represented by a totem. For example, Spring is associated with the East, where the sun rises, and signifies seeing things in new ways; its totem is the Eagle. The four

Prize totem
A chief or warrior of the Fox tribe affirmed his rank with this bear claw necklace.

Directional totems are explained on pp.18–19. Your *Elemental totem* relates to your instinctive behaviours. The qualities of the four Elements – Fire, Water, Earth, and Air – and their totems are introduced on pp.20–21.

THREE AFFINITIES

Each birth time also has an affinity with a tree, a stone, and a colour (see pp.36–41). These three affinities have qualities that can strengthen you during challenging times.

"If a man is to succeed, he must be governed not by his inclination, but by an understanding of the ways of animals..." Teton Sioux teaching

THE TWELVE
BIRTH TOTEMS

THE TWELVE BIRTH TIMES ARE REPRESENTED BY TOTEMS,
EACH ONE AN ANIMAL THAT BEST EXPRESSES THE
QUALITIES INHERENT IN THAT BIRTH TIME.

Earth Medicine associates an animal totem with each birth time (the two sets of dates below reflect the difference in season between the northern and southern hemispheres). These animals help to connect you to the powers and abilities that they represent. For an in-depth study of the Wolf birth totem, see pp.28–29.

FALCON
21 March–19 April (N. Hem)
22 Sept–22 Oct (S. Hem)
Falcons are full of initiative, but often rush in to make decisions they may later regret. Lively and extroverted, they have enthusiasm for new experiences but can sometimes lack persistence.

DEER
21 May–20 June (N. Hem)
23 Nov–21 Dec (S. Hem)
Deer are willing to sacrifice the old for the new. They loathe routine, thriving on variety and challenges. They have a wild side, often leaping from one situation or relationship into another without reflection.

BEAVER
20 April–20 May (N. Hem)
23 Oct–22 Nov (S. Hem)
Practical and steady, Beavers have a capacity for perseverance. Good homemakers, they are warm and affectionate but need harmony and peace to avoid becoming irritable. They have a keen aesthetic sense.

WOODPECKER
21 June–21 July (N. Hem)
22 Dec–19 Jan (S. Hem)
Emotional and sensitive, Woodpeckers are warm to those closest to them, and willing to sacrifice their needs for those of their loved ones. They have lively imaginations but can be worriers.

SALMON
22 July–21 August (N. Hem)
20 Jan–18 Feb (S. Hem)
Enthusiastic and self-confident, Salmon people enjoy running things. They are uncompromising and forceful, and can occasionally seem a little arrogant or self-important. They are easily hurt by neglect.

OWL
23 Nov–21 Dec (N. Hem)
21 May–20 June (S. Hem)
Owls need freedom of expression. They are lively, self-reliant, and have an eye for detail. Inquisitive and adaptable, they have a tendency to overextend themselves. Owls are often physically courageous.

BROWN BEAR
22 August–21 Sept (N. Hem)
19 Feb–20 March (S. Hem)
Brown Bears are hardworking, practical, and self-reliant. They do not like change, preferring to stick to what is familiar. They have a flair for fixing things, are good-natured, and make good friends.

GOOSE
22 Dec–19 Jan (N. Hem)
21 June–21 July (S. Hem)
Goose people are far-sighted idealists who are willing to explore the unknown. They approach life with enthusiasm, determined to fulfil their dreams. They are perfectionists, and can appear unduly serious.

CROW
22 Sept–22 Oct (N. Hem)
21 March–19 April (S. Hem)
Crows dislike solitude and feel most comfortable in company. Although usually pleasant and good-natured, they can be strongly influenced by negative atmospheres, becoming gloomy and prickly.

OTTER
20 Jan–18 Feb (N. Hem)
22 July–21 August (S. Hem)
Otters are friendly, lively, and perceptive. They feel inhibited by too many rules and regulations, which often makes them appear eccentric. They like cleanliness and order, and have original minds.

SNAKE
23 Oct–22 Nov (N. Hem)
20 April–20 May (S. Hem)
Snakes are secretive and mysterious, hiding their feelings beneath a cool exterior. Adaptable, determined, and imaginative, they are capable of bouncing back from tough situations encountered in life.

WOLF
19 Feb–20 March (N. Hem)
22 August–21 Sept (S. Hem)
Wolves are sensitive, artistic, and intuitive – people to whom others turn for help. They value freedom and their own space, and are easily affected by others. They are philosophical, trusting, and genuine.

THE INFLUENCE OF THE
DIRECTIONS

ALSO KNOWN BY NATIVE AMERICANS AS THE FOUR
WINDS, THE INFLUENCE OF THE FOUR DIRECTIONS IS
EXPERIENCED THROUGH YOUR INNER SENSES.

Regarded as the "keepers" or "caretakers" of the Universe, the four Directions or alignments were also referred to by Native Americans as the four Winds because their presence was felt rather than seen.

DIRECTIONAL TOTEMS

In Earth Medicine, each Direction or Wind is associated with a season and a time of day. Thus the Winter birth times – Renewal time, Cleansing time, and Blustery Winds time –

all fall within the North Direction, and night. The Direction to which your birth time belongs influences the nature of your inner senses.

The East Direction is associated with illumination. Its totem is the Eagle – a bird that soars close to the Sun and can see clearly from height. The South is the Direction of Summer and the afternoon. It signifies growth and fruition, fluidity, and emotions. Its totem, the Mouse, symbolizes productivity, feelings, and an ability to perceive detail.

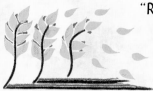

"Remember...the circle of the sky, the stars, the supernatural Winds breathing night and day...the four Directions." Pawnee teaching

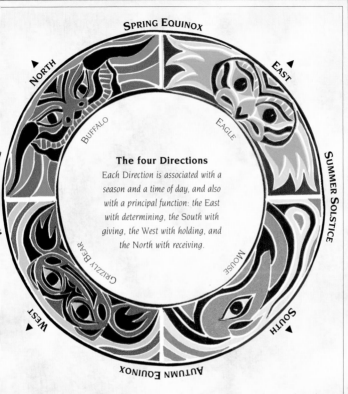

SPRING EQUINOX

NORTH

EAST

SUMMER SOLSTICE

BUFFALO

EAGLE

The four Directions

Each Direction is associated with a season and a time of day, and also with a principal function: the East with determining, the South with giving, the West with holding, and the North with receiving.

GRIZZLY BEAR

MOUSE

WEST

SOUTH

AUTUMN EQUINOX

The West is the Direction of Autumn and the evening. It signifies transformation – from day to night, from Summer to Winter – and the qualities of introspection and conservation. Its totem is the Grizzly Bear, which represents strength drawn from within. The North is the Direction of Winter and the night, and is associated with the mind and its sustenance – knowledge. Its totem is the Buffalo, an animal that was honoured by Native Americans as the great material "provider".

THE INFLUENCE OF THE ELEMENTS

THE FOUR ELEMENTS – AIR, FIRE, WATER, AND EARTH –
PERVADE EVERYTHING AND INDICATE THE NATURE OF
MOVEMENT AND THE ESSENCE OF WHO YOU ARE.

Elements are intangible qualities that describe the essential state or character of all things. In Earth Medicine, the four Elements are allied with four fundamental modes of activity and are associated with different aspects of the self. Air expresses free movement in all directions; it is related to the mind and to thinking. Fire indicates expansive motion; it is linked with the spirit and with intuition. Water signifies fluidity; it

Elemental profile
The Elemental configuration of Wolf is Water of Air. Air is the Principal Element and Water the Elemental Aspect.

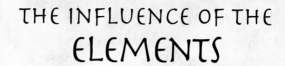

WATER

AIR

EARTH

FIRE

AIR

EARTH

has associations with the soul and the emotions. Earth symbolizes stability; it is related to the physical body and the sensations.

ELEMENTAL DISTRIBUTION

On the Medicine Wheel one Element is associated with each of the four Directions – Fire in the East, Earth in the West, Air in the North, and Water in the South. These are known as the Principal Elements.

FIRE

EARTH

AIR

WATER

The four Elements also have an individual association with each of the twelve birth times – known as the Elemental Aspects. They follow a cyclical sequence around the Wheel based on the action of the Sun (Fire) on the Earth, producing atmosphere (Air) and condensation (Water).

The three birth times that share an Elemental Aspect belong to the same Elemental family or "clan", with a totem that gives insight into its key characteristics. Wolf people belong to the Frog clan (see pp.34–35).

ELEMENTAL EMPHASIS

For each birth time, the qualities of the Elemental Aspect usually predominate over those of the Principal Element, although both are present to give a specific configuration, such as Fire of Earth (for Wolf's, see pp.34–35). For Falcon, Woodpecker, and Otter, the Principal Element and the Elemental Aspect are identical (for example, Air of Air), so people of these totems tend to express that Element intensely.

THE INFLUENCE OF THE MOON

THE WAXING AND WANING OF THE MOON DURING ITS FOUR PHASES HAS A CRUCIAL INFLUENCE ON THE FORMATION OF PERSONALITY AND HUMAN ENDEAVOUR.

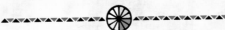

Native Americans regarded the Sun and Moon as indicators respectively of the active and receptive energies inherent in Nature (see p.24), as well as the measurers of time. They associated solar influences with conscious activity and the exercise of reason and the will, and lunar influences with subconscious activity and the emotional and intuitive aspects of human nature.

The Waxing Moon

This phase lasts for approximately eleven days. It is a time of growth and therefore ideal for developing new ideas and concentrating your efforts into new projects.

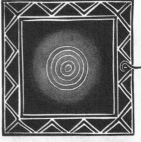

The Full Moon

Lasting about three days, this is when lunar power is at its height. It is therefore a good time for completing what was developed during the Waxing Moon.

THE FOUR PHASES

There are four phases in the twenty-nine-day lunar cycle, each one an expression of energy reflecting a particular mode of activity. They can be likened to the phases of growth of a flowering plant through the seasons: the emergence of buds (Waxing Moon), the bursting of flowers (Full Moon), the falling away of flowers (Waning Moon), and the germination of seeds (Dark Moon). The influence of each phase can be felt in two ways: in the formation of personality and in day-to-day life.

The energy expressed by the phase of the Moon at the time of your birth has a strong influence on personality. For instance, someone born during the Dark Moon is likely to be inward-looking, whilst a person born during the Full Moon may be more expressive. Someone born during a Waxing Moon is likely to have an outgoing nature, whilst a person born during a Waning Moon may be reserved. Consult a set of Moon tables to discover the phase the Moon was in on *your* birthday.

In your day-to-day life, the benefits of coming into harmony with the Moon's energies are considerable. Experience the energy of the four phases by consciously working with them. A Native American approach is described below.

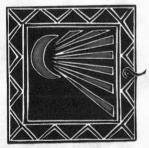

The Waning Moon

A time for making changes, this phase lasts for an average of eleven days. Use it to improve and modify, and to dispose of what is no longer needed or wanted.

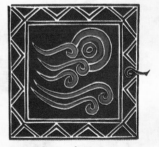

The Dark Moon

The Moon disappears from the sky for around four days. This is a time for contemplation of what has been achieved, and for germinating the seeds for the new.

23

THE INFLUENCE OF
ENERGY FLOW

THE MEDICINE WHEEL REFLECTS THE PERFECT BALANCE OF THE COMPLEMENTARY ACTIVE AND RECEPTIVE ENERGIES THAT CO-EXIST IN NATURE.

E nergy flows through Nature in two complementary ways, which can be expressed in terms of active and receptive, or male and female. The active energy principle is linked with the Elements of Fire and Air, and the receptive principle with Water and Earth.

Each of the twelve birth times has an active or receptive energy related to its Elemental Aspect. Travelling around the Wheel, the two energies alternate with each birth time, resulting in an equal balance of active and receptive energies, as in Nature.

Active energy is associated with the Sun and conscious activity. Those whose birth times take this principle prefer to pursue experience. They are conceptual,

energetic, outgoing, practical, and analytical. Receptive energy is associated with the Moon and subconscious activity. Those whose birth times take this principle prefer to attract experience. They are intuitive, reflective, conserving, emotional, and nurturing.

THE WAKAN-TANKA

At the heart of the Wheel lies an S-shape within a circle, the symbol of the life-giving source of everything that comes into physical existence – seemingly out of nothing. Named by the Plains Indians as Wakan-Tanka (Great Power), it can also be perceived as energy coming into form and form reverting to energy in the unending continuity of life.

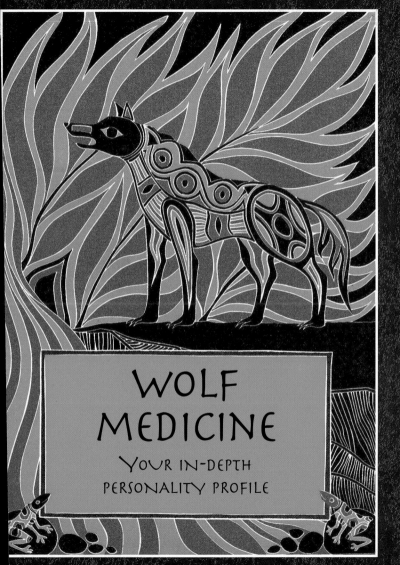

WOLF
MEDICINE

YOUR IN-DEPTH
PERSONALITY PROFILE

SEASON OF BIRTH
BLUSTERY WINDS TIME

THE TURBULENT NATURE OF WINTER CAN BE FELT IN THE
THIRD BIRTH TIME OF THE SEASON, LENDING THOSE BORN
THEN PASSIONATE SENSITIVITY AND ADAPTABILITY.

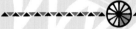

Blustery Winds time is one of the twelve birth times, the fundamental division of the year into twelve seasonal segments (see pp.12–13). As the third period of the Winter cycle, it is the time of the year when the winds are turbulent and the temperature warm enough to melt the last of the snow and ice, in readiness for the new growth of the Spring.

INFLUENCE OF NATURE
The qualities and characteristics imbued in Nature at this time form the basis of your own nature. So, just

as the winds are gusty, constantly changing direction, so, if you were born during Blustery Winds time, you have a passionate but adaptable nature. You are able to focus your considerable energies in seemingly opposing directions at the same time, and you have the emotional resilience to recover quickly from any disappointments you encounter.

Your compassionate, generous nature fully matches the benevolence and hopefulness of the season, which anticipates the warmth of Spring. As Nature begins to emerge renewed but still sleepy after the purification of Winter, so you possess the heightened awareness of one energized after sleep but whose mind is still partially in the world of dreams. This makes you highly intuitive and sensitive to the true opinions and feelings of others. Consequently you tend to rely on intuition rather than logic when faced with a problem.

STAGE OF LIFE

This time of year might be compared to the maturity of the later years in life. In human development terms, it is a period in which worldly ambitions and practical issues are of less importance than the desire to determine the purpose or meaning of life. It is a time of thoughtful reflection and intuitive insights into philosophical and spiritual matters, and of concern for the well-being of others.

ACHIEVE YOUR POTENTIAL

Your sensitive and intuitive nature means that you are readily able to understand the essence of a situation or person. Your sympathetic

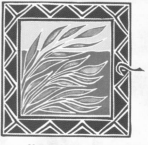

Nature's energy

Nature brings to a close its austere phase in this, the last cycle of Winter before the Spring equinox. Warmer temperatures defrost the Earth, and gusty winds drive rain into the soil, ready for planting.

approach makes you highly popular with others in times of stress and confusion. You are likely, however, to be adversely affected by the troubled emotions of others and may also find yourself unappreciated by some you have helped. Cleanse yourself from such negativity, and recover your energies by periodically spending some time on your own. Also, try to avoid mistaking criticism of your work for criticism of yourself. Stand back from your creations.

"Life is a circle from childhood to childhood; so it is with everything where power moves." Black Elk teaching

BIRTH TOTEM
THE WOLF

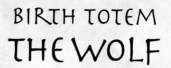

THE ESSENTIAL NATURE AND CHARACTERISTIC
BEHAVIOUR OF THE WOLF EXPRESSES THE PERSONALITY
TYPE OF THOSE BORN DURING BLUSTERY WINDS TIME.

Like the wolf, people born during Blustery Winds time are intuitive, loyal, compassionate, and protective. If you were born at this time, you have a warm, sensitive, romantic, philosophical, and adaptable nature that seeks to discover the true meaning or purpose of life.

Emotional, perceptive, and gentle, you often act instinctively rather than logically, and, in times of difficulty, are always ready to offer sympathy and understanding to friends and colleagues, who rely on you for emotional support. Unfortunately, your natural empathy means you tend to absorb others' negative feelings, which can leave you emotionally drained.

Wolf power
Warm and intuitive, the wolf also expresses the protective aspect of those born at this time.

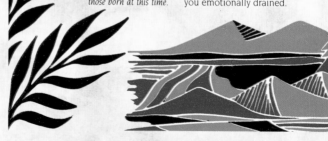

Trusting and unworldly, you are devoted to those close to you and can be easily hurt by those you love. Creative and sensitive, you have a highly developed aesthetic sense, and identify strongly with your creative or artistic endeavours, often perceiving criticism of your work as a personal attack.

HEALTH MATTERS

Although drawn to natural remedies and preventative medicine, you enjoy food and drink, and tend to over-eat. You are therefore prone to unhealthy weight gain, circulatory problems, and high blood pressure.

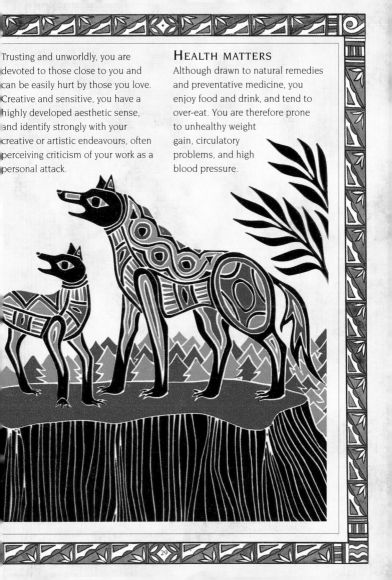

THE WOLF AND
RELATIONSHIPS

SENSITIVE AND INTUITIVE, WOLF PEOPLE ARE CARING
FRIENDS. THEY MAKE WARM, LOVING PARTNERS BUT FIND
THEIR OWN STRONG EMOTIONS DIFFICULT TO HANDLE.

Valued for their compassion and understanding, Wolf people can be counted on to offer insight and sympathy. Like their totem animal, they are intuitive and often see beneath surface signs to the truth. If your birth totem is Wolf, you empathize strongly with other people. However, your great sensitivity means you absorb their problems like a sponge. Try to treat yourself with equal compassion. You need time alone to recharge your batteries or you will feel drained.

LOVING RELATIONSHIPS
Romantic Wolf people have a great need for love and affection, but their desire for closeness may be at odds with their love of freedom. Male Wolf is caring but often idolizes his lover, while female Wolf is warm and

sensitive. Both are gentle lovers who need a responsive partner.

Problems usually stem from your oversensitivity to criticism; you tend to take things too personally. You also find the strength of your own feelings disturbing and may try to suppress them, making your partner confused. Try to temper your emotions with discernment and sound judgement.

COPING WITH WOLF
Wolf people are strongly instinctive, so never betray their confidence or you will lose their trust. They must be able to make their own choices; don't pressure them, but let them act freely from their own intuition, or they will become frustrated and bitter. Handle Wolf people with kindness, love, and consideration if you want to earn their affection and trust.

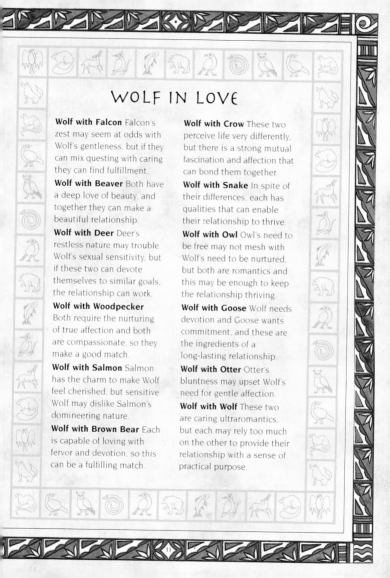

WOLF IN LOVE

Wolf with Falcon Falcon's zest may seem at odds with Wolf's gentleness, but if they can mix questing with caring they can find fulfillment.

Wolf with Beaver Both have a deep love of beauty, and together they can make a beautiful relationship.

Wolf with Deer Deer's restless nature may trouble Wolf's sexual sensitivity, but if these two can devote themselves to similar goals, the relationship can work.

Wolf with Woodpecker Both require the nurturing of true affection and both are compassionate, so they make a good match.

Wolf with Salmon Salmon has the charm to make Wolf feel cherished, but sensitive Wolf may dislike Salmon's domineering nature.

Wolf with Brown Bear Each is capable of loving with fervor and devotion, so this can be a fulfilling match.

Wolf with Crow These two perceive life very differently, but there is a strong mutual fascination and affection that can bond them together.

Wolf with Snake In spite of their differences, each has qualities that can enable their relationship to thrive.

Wolf with Owl Owl's need to be free may not mesh with Wolf's need to be nurtured, but both are romantics and this may be enough to keep the relationship thriving.

Wolf with Goose Wolf needs devotion and Goose wants commitment, and these are the ingredients of a long-lasting relationship.

Wolf with Otter Otter's bluntness may upset Wolf's need for gentle affection.

Wolf with Wolf These two are caring ultraromantics, but each may rely too much on the other to provide their relationship with a sense of practical purpose.

DIRECTIONAL TOTEM
THE BUFFALO

THE BUFFALO SYMBOLIZES THE INFLUENCE OF THE NORTH ON WOLF PEOPLE, WHOSE STRONG POWERS OF INTUITION COMPLEMENT THEIR INNATE WISDOM.

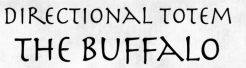

Renewal time, Cleansing time, and Blustery Winds time all fall within the quarter of the Medicine Wheel associated with the North Direction or Wind.

The North is aligned with Winter and with night, and it is therefore associated with patience, the hidden energy that lies beneath the surface, purity, and renewal. It is likened to the preparation for new life and new ideas – the reflective stillness that precedes rebirth and the time of rapid growth. The power of the North's influence is primarily with the mind and wisdom, and its principal function is the power of sustenance. It takes as its totem the revered and life-sustaining buffalo.

Buffalo skull
This Blackfeet-painted buffalo skull represents the buffalo, which is associated with sustenance of mind and body.

The specific influence of the North on Wolf people is on intuitive sense, enabling you to divine hidden truths, and endowing you with a deep sensitivity both to people's feelings and to mystical matters. It has associations with the Moon – your creative powers may wax and wane according to its cycle. It also gives you a deep thirst for wisdom.

BUFFALO CHARACTERISTICS
Of all animals, the buffalo was most revered by Native Americans because many tribes depended on it for their survival. Every part of it was

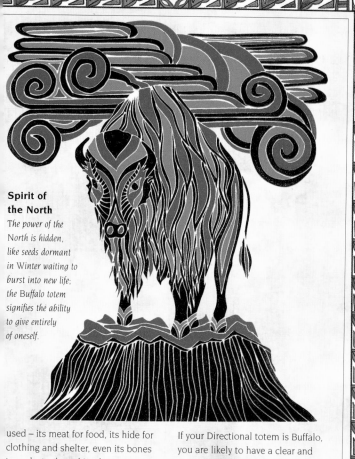

Spirit of the North

The power of the North is hidden, like seeds dormant in Winter waiting to burst into new life; the Buffalo totem signifies the ability to give entirely of oneself.

used – its meat for food, its hide for clothing and shelter, even its bones to make tools and implements – so it was said to symbolize the spirit that gives completely of itself.

If your Directional totem is Buffalo, you are likely to have a clear and keen mind, a quiet wisdom, and the power of renewing your energies from your own inner resources.

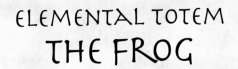

ELEMENTAL TOTEM
THE FROG

LIKE THE FROG, WHICH SENSES EVERY RIPPLE IN THE
WATER, WOLF PEOPLE'S INTUITIVE NATURE AND
EMOTIONAL SENSITIVITY REQUIRES FREE REIN.

The Elemental Aspect of Wolf people is Water. They share this Aspect with Woodpecker and Snake people, who all therefore belong to the same Elemental family or "clan" (see pp.20–21 for an introduction to the influence of the Elements). Each Elemental clan has a totem to provide insight into its essential characteristics.

THE FROG CLAN

The totem of the Elemental clan of Water is Frog, which symbolizes a sensitive, emotional, thoughtful, and intuitive nature.

The frog is at home both in water and on land, diving below the surface then sitting still, attuned to every movement around it. So, if you belong to this clan, you have the ability to adapt, while your intuition enables you to see beneath surface

Below the surface
The frog symbolizes the fundamental quality of Water: deep sensitivity.

appearances and to understand the moods of others.

Imaginative, responsive, and intense, you have deep emotions which you "bottle up" at times. You dislike feeling vulnerable and can be secretive. You crave understanding and true freedom to express yourself both creatively and emotionally.

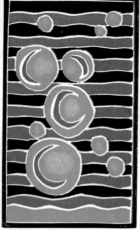

Water of Air

The Element of Water feeds Air, generating sensitivity and strong clarity of mind.

may sometimes find yourself in situations where you feel you are pulling in two directions at once. This can make you feel frustrated and lead to self-doubt. At times like these, or when you are feeling stressed or are facing a dilemma, try this soothing exercise. Find a quiet spot near water – with which you have a natural affinity – by a river or lake, the sea or a pool, away from the polluting effects of traffic and the activities of others.

ELEMENTAL PROFILE

For Wolf people, the predominant Elemental Aspect of emotional Water is fundamentally affected by the qualities of your Principal Element – clarifying Air. So, if you were born at this time, you are likely to have an abundance of creativity and sensitivity together with a clear mind and questing intellect, balancing your powerful emotions with clarity of thought and vision.

You may have a tendency to be indecisive, driven by the turbulence of Water and the urge to change that is inherent in Air. Consequently, you

Simply enjoy the play of light or reflections on the surface and let the sound of the water wash over you as you breathe slowly and deeply. With each in-breath, feel the energizing power of the life-force course through you, bringing you the clarity of a mountain stream, and refreshing your body, mind, and spirit.

STONE AFFINITY
JADE

By using the gemstone with which your own essence resonates, you can tap into the power of the Earth itself and awaken your inner strengths.

Gemstones are minerals that are formed within the Earth itself in an exceedingly slow but continuous process. Native Americans valued them not only for their beauty but also for being literally part of the Earth, and therefore possessing part of its life-force.

They regarded gemstones as being "alive" – channellers of energy that could be used in many ways: to heal, to protect, or for meditation.

Every gemstone has a different energy or vibration. On the Medicine Wheel, a stone is associated with each birth time, the energy of which

Polished jade

Sometimes known as the "dream stone", jade was believed to help you interpret your dreams.

resonates with the essence of those born during that time. Because of this energy affiliation, your stone can help bring you into harmony with the Earth and create balance within yourself. It can enhance and develop your good qualities and endow you with the abilities you need.

ENERGY RESONANCE

Wolf people have an affinity with jade, a fine-grained stone which occurs in many colours; the most prized type is deep emerald-green imperial jade. It is especially tough, making it an inspirational emblem

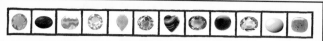

ACTIVATE YOUR GEMSTONE

Obtain a piece of jade and cleanse it by holding it under cold running water. Allow it to dry naturally, then, holding the stone with both hands, bring it up to your mouth and blow into it sharply and hard three or four times in order to impregnate it with your breath. Next, hold it firmly in one hand and silently welcome it into your life as a friend and helper.

When you want to boost your self-esteem or need help in transforming your dreams into reality, use your jade as an aid to meditation. Find a quiet spot to sit without fear of interruption and hold the jade in your left hand, which receives subtle energies. Focus on the stone and ask for guidance in discovering how best to use your abilities. Listen for the still, small voice of your inner self.

for Wolf people who are highly sensitive. Native Americans often carried jade as a talisman to attract good fortune. They associated it with wisdom and clarity, and it was said to promote a long and fruitful life.

If your birth totem is Wolf, you will find jade a valuable aid in helping you realize your dreams and aspirations and create tangible results. It is believed to ground higher energies and inspire

achievement, making it a powerful totem for you at times when you need to root your spiritual and intuitive nature in practical realities.

Jade power
To benefit most from its effect, wear or carry jade, and keep some at home to create a sense of peace.

"The outline of the stone is round; the power of the stone is endless." Lakota Sioux teaching

TREE AFFINITY
OAK

GAIN A DEEPER UNDERSTANDING OF YOUR OWN NATURE
AND AWAKEN POWERS LYING DORMANT WITHIN YOU BY
RESPECTING AND CONNECTING WITH YOUR AFFINITY TREE.

rees have an important part to play in the protection of Nature's mechanisms and in the maintenance of the Earth's atmospheric balance, which is essential for the survival of the human race.

Native Americans referred to trees as "Standing People" because they stand firm, obtaining strength from their connection with the Earth. They therefore teach us the importance of being grounded, whilst at the same time listening to, and reaching for, our higher

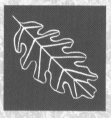

aspirations. When respected as living beings, trees can provide insight into the workings of Nature and our own inner selves.

On the Medicine Wheel, each birth time is associated with a particular kind of tree, the basic qualities of which complement the nature of those born during that time. Wolf people have an affinity with the oak. Prized for its great size and durability, the oak is a potent symbol of strength and achievement. Like the sturdy oak, Wolf stands firm when all around is in turmoil, a

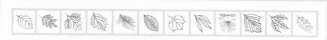

CONNECT WITH YOUR TREE

Appreciate the beauty of your affinity tree and study its nature carefully, for it has an affinity with your own nature.

The mighty oak tree has a wide trunk, very deep roots, and deeply lobed leaves. Held sacred in ancient times, the oak is still valued for its great strength and durability; the wood was much used in shipbuilding, and the bark for tanning leather.

Try the following exercise when you need to revitalize your inner strength. Stand beside your affinity tree. Place the palms of your hands on its trunk and rest your forehead on the backs of your hands. Inhale slowly and experience energy from the tree's roots flow through your body. If easily available, obtain a cutting or twig from your affinity tree to keep as a totem or helper.

steadfast support to others in a crisis. However, this can drain Wolf's reserves of strength and vitality. When Wolf people feel depleted by outside negativity, they can tap into their own powers of self-renewal and inner strength by connecting with their tree (see panel above).

THE POWER OF PATIENCE

If your birth totem is Wolf, you are intuitive and compassionate with deep emotions, but you can be indecisive and something of a dreamer, which can prevent you from realizing your true potential.

Just as it grows slowly from a tiny acorn into the sturdiest of trees, the oak is an expression of the power of patience in the pursuit of worthwhile goals. When the fulfilment of your ambitions seems a far-off dream, draw on the energy of the oak; its steadfastness will help you find your strength and discover that from small beginnings grow great achievements.

"All healing plants are given by Wakan-Tanka; therefore they are holy." Lakota Sioux teaching

COLOUR AFFINITY
BLUE-GREEN

ENHANCE YOUR POSITIVE QUALITIES BY USING THE
POWER OF YOUR AFFINITY COLOUR TO AFFECT YOUR
EMOTIONAL AND MENTAL STATES.

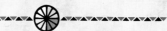

Each birth time has an affinity with a particular colour. This is the colour that resonates best with the energies of the people born during that time. Exposure to your affinity colour will encourage a positive emotional and mental response, while exposure to colours that clash with your affinity colour will have a negative effect on your sense of well-being.

Blue-green resonates with Wolf people. Blue is associated with spirituality and intuitive wisdom and green with Nature and gradual growth. Blue is the colour of compassion and tranquillity, and freedom of

Colour scheme

*Let a blue-green colour theme be the
thread that runs through your home,
from the table settings to
the walls and floors.*

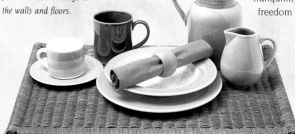

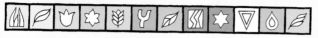

BATHE IN YOUR COLOUR

Pour a few drops of blue and green aromatherapy oil into a bath of warm water. Gently disturb the water to disperse the oil, before climbing in. When you are ready, submerge your body in the water. Make sure you have at least half an hour to spare, so you can indulge in a relaxed, unhurried soaking.

Bathing in your colour will release tension, relieve stress, and leave your skin feeling soft and smooth. It is especially beneficial if you are feeling emotionally or mentally drained, or depressed. Allow any thoughts and sensations to flow through your mind and body, and reflect on them.

movement and ideas, while green suggests warmth and development within form. Blue-green therefore embodies calm discrimination, harmonious creativity, and the love of both truth and beauty.

COLOUR BENEFITS

Strengthen your aura and enhance your positive qualities by introducing shades of blue and green to the interior decor of your home. Spots of colour can make all the difference. A blue-green tinted lampshade, for example, can alter the ambience of a room, or try placing an aquamarine-patterned rug on the floor, or blue and green patterned cushions on the sofa.

If you need a confidence boost, wear something that contains blue-green. Whenever your energies are low, practise the colour bathing exercise outlined above, to balance your emotions, awaken your creativity, and help you to feel joyful.

"The power of the spirit should be honoured with its colour." Lakota Sioux teaching

WORKING THE WHEEL
LIFE PATH

Consider your birth profile as a starting point in the development of your character and the achievement of personal fulfilment.

Each of the twelve birth times is associated with a particular path of learning, or with a collection of lessons to be learned through life. By following your path of learning you will develop strengths in place of weaknesses, achieve a greater sense of harmony with the world, and discover inner peace.

YOUR PATH OF LEARNING
For Wolf people, the first lesson on your path of learning is to accept that

changes are an inevitable part of life. Because of your highly emotional relationship with every aspect of your life, whenever you are confronted by change, however small, you are filled with anxiety out of all proportion to the actual impact of it on your life. Try to perceive beginnings and endings as part of a continuous process of personal development rather than a threat to

"Each man's road is shown to him within his own heart. There he sees all the truths of life." *Cheyenne teaching*

your entire well-being. Your innate adaptability will ensure that you benefit from any changes.

Wolf people also need to try to overcome indecisiveness and vagueness. Because you operate intuitively rather than rationally and because you are so susceptible to the influence of the feelings of those around you, it is often difficult for you to discern the best course to take. When you next need to make an important decision, find time to separate yourself from those close to you, so that you can hear your own inner voice.

Your third lesson is to learn to be more discriminating about those you support emotionally. Sensitive and compassionate, you are invaluable to others in times of crisis. But, if you try to help everyone, you will find yourself completely drained of emotional energy. Try to identify those who really need your help, and focus your energies on them.

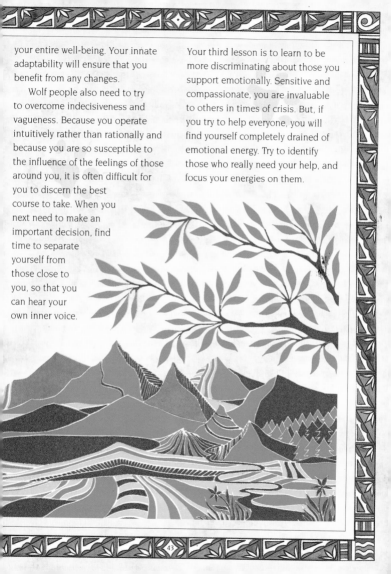

WORKING THE WHEEL
MEDICINE POWER

HARNESS THE POWERS OF OTHER BIRTH TIMES TO TRANSFORM YOUR WEAKNESSES INTO STRENGTHS AND MEET THE CHALLENGES IN YOUR LIFE.

The whole spectrum of human qualities and abilities is represented on the Medicine Wheel. The totems and affinities associated with each birth time indicate the basic qualities with which those born at that time are equipped.

Study your path of learning (see pp.42–43) to identify those aspects of your personality that may need to be strengthened, then look at other birth times to discover the totems and affinities that can assist you in this task. For example, your Elemental profile is Water of Air (see pp.34–35), so for balance you need the enthusiasm of Fire and the

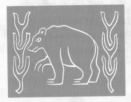

Complementary affinity

A key strength of Brown Bear – weak in Wolf – is the ability to maintain a sense of identity.

stabilizing qualities of Earth. Beaver's Elemental profile is Earth of Fire and Owl's is Fire of Earth, so meditate on these birth totems. In addition, you may find it useful to study the profiles of the other two members of your Elemental clan of Frog – Woodpecker and Snake – to discover how the same Elemental Aspect can be expressed differently.

Also helpful is the birth totem that sits opposite yours on the Medicine Wheel, which contains qualities that complement or enhance your own. This is known as your complementary affinity, which for Wolf people is Brown Bear.

ESSENTIAL STRENGTHS

Described below are the essential strengths of each birth totem. To develop a quality that is weak in yourself or that you need to meet a particular challenge, meditate upon the birth totem that contains the attribute you need. Obtain a representation of the relevant totem – a claw, tooth, or feather; a picture, ring, or model. Affirm that the power it represents is within you.

Falcon medicine is the power of keen observation and the ability to act decisively and energetically whenever action is required.

Beaver medicine is the ability to think creatively and laterally – to develop alternative ways of doing or thinking about things.

Deer medicine is characterized by sensitivity to the intentions of others and to that which might be detrimental to your well-being.

Woodpecker medicine is the ability to establish a steady rhythm throughout life and to be tenacious in protecting all that you hold dear.

Salmon medicine is the strength to be determined and courageous in the choice of goals you want to achieve and to have enough stamina to see a task through to the end.

Brown Bear medicine is the ability to be resourceful, hardworking, and dependable in times of need, and to draw on inner strength.

Crow medicine is the ability to transform negative or non-productive situations into positive ones and to transcend limitations.

Snake medicine is the talent to adapt easily to changes in circumstances and to manage transitional phases well.

Owl medicine is the power to see clearly during times of uncertainty and to conduct life consistently, according to long-term plans.

Goose medicine is the courage to do whatever might be necessary to protect your ideals and adhere to your principles in life.

Otter medicine is the ability to connect with your inner child, to be innovative and idealistic, and to thoroughly enjoy the ordinary tasks and routines of everyday life.

Wolf medicine is the courage to act according to your intuition and instincts rather than your intellect, and to be compassionate.

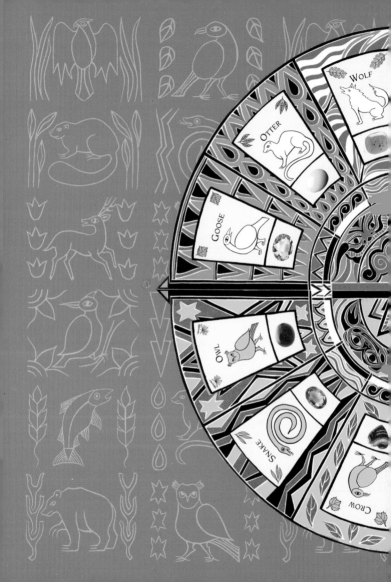